THE

SIDES OF THE BODY,

AND

DRUG-AFFINITIES.

HOMŒOPATHIC EXERCISES.

BY

Dr. C. von BŒNNINGHAUSEN,

Real, Honorary and Corresponding Member of the Homœopathic Societies of Paris, Madrid London, Palermo, Philadelphia, Rio de Janeiro, and of several literary and scientific Societies, &c.

EDITED BY

CHARLES J. HEMPEL, M. D.,

Fellow and Corresponding Member of the Pennsylvania Homœopathic College, Honorary Member of the Hahnemann Society of London, &c.

PHILADELPHIA:

PUBLISHED BY RADEMACHER & SHEEK, 239 ARCH STREET.

NEW YORK:—WILLIAM RADDE, 322 BROADWAY.

ST. LOUIS:—J. G. WESSELHŒFT, 79 MARKET STREET.

NEW ORLEANS:—D. R. LUYTIES, M. D.

1854.

THE SIDES OF THE BODY, AND DRUG-AFFINITIES.

HOMŒOPATHIC EXERCISES.

BY

Dr. C. von BŒNNINGHAUSEN,

Real, Honorary and Corresponding Member of the Homœopathic Societies of Paris, Madrid, London, Palermo, Philadelphia, Rio de Janeiro, and of several literary and scientific Societies, &c.

EDITED BY

CHARLES J. HEMPEL, M. D.,

Fellow and Corresponding Member of the Pennsylvania Homœopathic College, Honorary Member of the Hahnemann Society of London, &c.

PHILADELPHIA:

PUBLISHED BY RADEMACHER & SHEEK, 239 ARCH STREET.

NEW YORK:—WILLIAM RADDE, 322 BROADWAY.

ST. LOUIS:—J. G. WESSELHŒFT, 79 MARKET STREET.

NEW ORLEANS:—D. R. LUYTIES, M. D.

1854.

KING & BAIRD, Printers.

PREFACE.

At the annual convention of the homœopathic physicians of the Rhenish Provinces and Westphalia, which was held at Düsseldorf on the 28th of July of the present year, the necessity of strictly individualising every case of disease, and of studying with a corresponding accuracy the characteristic symptoms and peculiarities of drugs, was discussed among a variety of other subjects. Unless we are intimately acquainted with the character of the symptoms, which, like the red thread in the ropes of the English Navy, runs through the whole pathogenesis of every single drug, the process of individualising the phenomena of disease would lose its real value, inasmuch as the practitioner would be deprived of the means of applying his remedies to the case before him with positive certainty and precision. It seems therefore of the utmost importance to carefully collect, examine and verify all the facts which, in one way or another, are capable of leading to this desirable knowledge of the natural morbid symptoms as well as the physiological effects of our drugs.

To accomplish this end I had, originally for my own use, perfected the subsequent arrangement concerning the characteristic action of drugs on the *right or left side of the body*, and in numerous cases, where the want of decisive symptoms rendered the selection of the proper remedy doubtful, I had derived great advantages from it. The members of the convention, to whom this arrangement was shown, expressed their entire approbation with my plan, which was considered superior to the existing homœopathic publications in which this subject is not treated with sufficient completeness; and all expressed a desire that this little work might be given to the press for the benefit of the profession generally.

This gave rise to the publication of the present pages, which are few in number, but full of deep significance, and which it has cost me a great deal of labor to achieve. Any one who will take the trouble to study the characteristic peculiarities of our drugs in the original provings on the healthy, will find, that the records of such peculiarities are exceedingly scanty, and that it is precisely in the provings of our polychrests, which are constantly used in daily practice, that this want of all accurate distinction between the right and left side of the body, although frequent mention is made of semi-lateral ailments, is principally perceptible. In order to increase my materials, and to obtain a confirmation of my statements and data by experience, it became necessary to consult my own cases of cure, as well as those of other practitioners, and to devote a considerable deal of time and labor to this business which I could not have accomplished if I had not had carefully-conducted records of diseases to refer to. In spite of all the care and attention which I have bestowed upon this execution of my plan, I am not sure that I may not have committed a mistake or an oversight, especially in regard to the remedies that are not much used in the practice. As regards the vast majority of my indications, especially as far as the more frequently used remedies are concerned, I believe I can safely say that no errors need be apprehended.

Most drugs having manifested their action more or less on either side of the body, both during the proving and during their use in disease, the great question is, on which side this action was more particularly manifest. This distinction as well as the degrees of this action seemed to me best indicated by different print. The same plan was pursued in my repertories of the anti-psoric and non-anti-psoric drugs, and the public seemed to be pleased with it. For the benefit of those who do not possess these repertories which are partly out of the market, or have been replaced by the later works of Jahr, Mueller, Possart, and others, I will state that I used four different kinds of type.

1. COMMON TYPE, like: Agar. Alum. Ang. Ant. tart. Aur. &c. under LEFT SIDE; this kind of type indicates the lowest degree of action.

2. CLARENDON, such as: **Acon. Amm. Anac.** &c.; this kind of print indicates the next higher degree of action.

3. ITALICS, such as: *Ambr. Amm. muv. Ant. crud.* &c.; this kind of print indicates the third degree, which is pretty thoroughly verified and confirmed by experience; and lastly

4. TITLE, such as: **Brom. Sep.** &c.; this is the highest and most distinguished degree.

It seems impossible that, in such an arrangement as this, incorrect statements should have occurred; on the other hand, the finding a remedy is facilitated by the alphabetical order which has uniformly been observed.

In the second part of this work, the drug-affinities, the remedies which belong to the lowest degree, have been omitted for the purpose of avoiding all unnecessary crowding of mere names, which would simply tend to embarrass the reader; the other three degrees have been distinguished by the same varieties of print as in the first part. This second part contains the result of the examination to which I have subjected, for a number of years past, my former labors in reference to the same subject, and which has convinced me that an excessive number of remedies rendered their proper application in disease so much more difficult.

In conclusion I need scarcely remark that both parts of this little work, should only be looked upon and used as means of *facilitating the selection* of the proper remedy, and that the homœopathic law *similia similibus* should always remain the supreme guide in the treatment of disease whenever the characteristic symptoms of the drug are indicated with sufficient clearness to enable us to decide that the spirit of the remedy which we select, is in harmony with the character of the disease.

MUENSTER, August 1853.

C. v. BŒNNINGHAUSEN.

SIDES OF THE BODY.

INTERNAL HEAD.

LEFT SIDE.

Acon. Agar. Alum. *Ambr.* **Amm.** *A. mur.* **Anac.** Ang. *Ant. crud.* Ant. tart. *Ap.* *Arg.* *Arn.* **Ars.** *Asaf.* *Asar.* Aur. Bar. Bell. Bism. Bor. *Bov.* **Brom.** **Bry.** Calad. *Calc.* Camph. Cann. Canth. *Caps.* **C. an.** C. veg. **Caust.** *Cham.* Chel. **Chin.** *Cic.* Cina. **Clem.** Cocc. Coff. **Colch.** *Coloc.* Con. **Creos.** *Croc.* **Cupr.** *Cycl.* *Dig.* Dros. **Dulc.** *Euph.* Euphr. Ferr. Fluor. *Graph.* *Guaj.* Hell. Hep. Hyosc. Ignat. *Jod.* **Ipec.** *Kali.* *Lach.* **Laur.** Led. Lyc. **M. Arct.** *M. austr.* *Magn.* **Mang.** Mar. **Men.** *Merc.* *Mezer.* Millef. Mosch. **M. ac.** Natr. N. mur. **Nitr.** *N. ac.* *N. mosch.* **N. vom.** *Oleand.* Op. *Par.* **Petr.** **Phosph.** **Ph. ac.** *Plat.* Plumb. *Psor.* **Puls.** R. bulb. R. scel. Rheum. *Rhod.* **Rhus.** Ruta. Sabad. **Sabin.** *Samb.* **Sassap.** Scill. S. corn. *Selen.* Seneg. **Sep.** Sil. *Spig.* **Spong.** **Stann.** **Staph.** Stram. Stront. *Sulph.* **S. ac.** *Tar.* Thuj. Valer. **Veratr.** Verb. V. od. Viol. tric. Vit. *Zinc.*

RIGHT SIDE.

Acon. **Agar.** *Alum.* Ambr. Amm. **A. mur.** Anac. Ang. Ant. crud. Ant. tart. **Ap.** Arg. **Arn.** Ars. **Asaf.** Asar. Aur. Bar. **Bell.** *Bism.* *Bor.* Bov. Brom. *Bry.* **Calad.** **Calc.** Camph. **Cann.** *Canth.* **Caps.** C. an. **C. veg.** *Caust.* **Cham.** *Chel.* Chin. Cic. *Cina.* Clem. Cocc. Coff. **Colch.** Coloc. Con. Creos. Croc. Cupr. Cycl. Dig. **Dros.** *Dulc.* Euph. Euphr. Ferr. *Fluor.* **Graph.** Guaj. **Hell.** *Hep.* **Hyosc.** **Ignat.** Jod. Kali. **Lach.** Laur. Led. *Lyc.* M. arct. M. austr. **Magn.** Mang. *Mar.* Men. Merc. Mezer. **Millef.** *Mosch.* M. ac. Natr. *N. mur.* Nitr. N. ac. **N. mosch.** *N. vom.* **Oleand.** Op. Par. Petr. **Phosph.** **Phosph. ac.** **Plat.** *Plumb.* Psor. **Puls.** *R. bulb.* **R. scel.** **Rheum.** **Rhod.** *Rhus.* **Ruta.** **Sabad.** *Sabin.* Samb. Sassap. **Scill.** S. corn. Selen. Seneg. **Sep.** **Sil.** **Spig.** Spong. Stann. *Staph.* **Stram.** **Stront.** **Sulph.** *S. ac.* Tar. *Thuj.* *Valer.* Veratr. *Verb.* Viol. od. Viol. tric. **Vit.** **Zinc.**

EXTERNAL HEAD.

LEFT SIDE.

Acon. Agar. Alum. **Ammon.** Anac. **Ang. Ant. crud. Ant. tart.** Arg. *Ars. Asar.* Aur. **Bar.** Bell. **Bor.** Calc. Caps. *C. an.* **C veg. Caust. Cham.** Chel. *Chin.* **Clem. Cocc. Coloc.** *Dig. Dulc.* **Euph.** *Graph.* **Hep.** Jod. Kali. Laur. **Lyc. Magn.** M. mur. Mang. Men. *Merc.* Millef. **M. ac.** Natr. *N. mur.* Nitr. N. ac. **Oleand. Petr.** *Phosph.* **Ph. ac. Plat. Rhod.** Rhus. **Ruta. Seneg.** Sep. **Sil. Spig.** Staph. Stront. *Sulph.* **Tar. Thuj. Verb.** V. tric. Zinc.

RIGHT SIDE.

Agar. **Alum. Ambr.** Amm. **A. mur.** *Anac.* Ang. **Aur. Bell.** Bor. Brom. *Bry.* **Calc. Canth.** Caps. C. an. C. veg. Caust. *Chel.* Chin. Clem. Coloc. **Con. Creos.** Dig. *Dros.* Graph. **Guaj.** Hep. **Jod.** *Kali.* Laur. **Led. Lyc.** M. mur. **Mang.** *Men.* Merc. **Mezer.** M. ac. **Natr.** N. mur. **Nitr.** *N. ac.* Petr. Phosph. Ph. ac. Plat. Psor. *Puls.* R. bulb. **R. scel.** Rhod. *Rhus.* **Sabad.** *Sassap. Sep. Sil.* Spig. **Spong.** Stann. *Staph.* Stront. Thuj. **Veratr.** V. tric. **Vit. Zinc.**

EYES.

Acon. **Agar.** Alum. Ambr. Amm. A. mur. Anac. **A. cr.** A. tart. *Ap.* **Arn.** *Ars. Asaf. Asar.* **Aur.** Bar. **Bell. Bor.** Bov. Brom. *Bry.* Calad. **Calc.** Camph. Canth. Caps. *C. an.* C. veg. *Caust. Chel. Chin.* Cina. **Clem.** Colch. **Con. Croc. Dros.** Euph. **Euphr.** Ferr. **Fluor. Hell. Hep.** Ignat. Jod. Kali. *Laur.* **Lyc. M. arct.** *M. austr.* **Magn.** Mar. **Men. Merc.** *Mezer. Millef.* M. ac. **N. mur.** Nitr. **N. ac.** *N. vom.* **Oleand. Op.** Par. Petr. **Phosph. Ph. ac.** Plat. *Plumb.*

Acon. Agar. **Alum.** Ambr. *Amm.* A. mur. Anac. Ang. A. cr. **A. tart.** Ap. **Arn. Ars. Asaf.** Asar. Aur. **Bar. Bell. Bism.** Bor. **Bov. Brom.** Bry. Calad. **Calc.** *Camph.* **Cann.** *Canth.* Caps. C. an. *C. veg.* **Caust. Cham.** Chel. Chin. *Cic.* Cina. *Clem.* Coff. **Colch. Coloc.** *Con.* **Creos.** *Croc.* **Cycl.** *Dig.* Dros. **Euph.** *Euphr.* **Ferr.** *Fluor.* **Graph. Guaj. Hep. Hyosc. Ignat.** Jod. *Kali.* Laur. **Led. Lyc.** M. art. M. austr. **M. mur.** *Mang.* **Mar.** *Merc.* Millef. **M. ac.** *Natr.*

LEFT SIDE.

Psor. *Puls.* R. bulb. R. scel. **Rheum.** Rhod. **Rhus. Ruta.** Sabad. **Sabin.** Sassap. *Scill.* **Selen.** Seneg. *Sep.* **Sil.** *Spig.* **Spong.** *Stann.* Staph. Stram. **Stront.** **Sulph.** S. ac. *Tar.* *Thuj.* Valer. Veratr. **V. od. V. tr. Zinc.**

RIGHT SIDE.

N. mur. *Nitr.* **N. ac. N. mosch.** N.vom. Oleand. *Par.* **Petr.** *Phosph.* Ph. ac. **Plat.** *Plumb.* **Psor. Puls.** **R. bulb.** *R. scel.* Rheum. *Rhod.* **Rhus.** Ruta. Sabad. Sassap. Scill. Selen. **Seneg. Sep. Sil. Spig.** Spong. Stann. *Staph.* Stram. **Sulph.** S. ac. Tar. Thuj. **Valer.** *Veratr.* V. tr. **Vit.** Zinc.

EARS.

Acon. Agar. Alum. **Ambr.** *Amm.* A. mur. **Anac.** Ang. A. cr. *Ap.* Arg. *Arn.* **Ars. Asaf.** Asar. *Aur.*, Bar. Bell. **Bism. Bor.** *Brom.* *Bry.* Calad. **Calc.** *Camph.* Cann. Canth. **Caps.** C. an. **C. veg.** **Caust.** Chel. Chin. Cic. Clem. Colch. Coloc. Con. **Creos.** Croc. Cupr. Cycl. Dig. Dros. *Dulc.* Euph. Euphr. Ferr. Fluor. **Graph.** **Guaj.** Hep. **Ignat.** Jod. Kali. Lach. *Laur.* Lyc. Mang. Mar. Men. *Merc.* *Mezer.* *Millef.* **M. ac.** Natr. N. mur. Nitr. **N. ac.** N. mosch. **Oleand. Par.** Petr. **Phosph.** Ph. ac. Plat. Plumb. *Psor.* **Puls.** R. bulb. R. scel. Rheum. **Rhod. Rhus.** Sabad. **Sabin.** Sassap. Scill. Selen. Seneg. **Sep.** Sil. **Spig.** Spong. **Stann.** *Staph.* **Sulph.** Tar. Thuj. Valer.

Acon. **Agar.** *Alum.* Ambr. Amm. *A. mur.* Anac. *Ang.* *A. crud.* Ap. Arg. Arn. Ars. Asaf. **Asar. Bar. Bell.** Bor. *Bov.* Brom. Bry. **Calad.** *Calc.* **Cann.** *Canth.* *C. an.* C. veg. **Caust. Cham.** *Chel.* Chin. **Cic.** Clem. **Cocc.** **Colch.** Coloc. **Con.** Creos. Croc. **Cupr. Cycl.** Dig. Dros. Dulc. Euph. Euphr. Ferr. **Fluor.** Graph. **Hell.** *Hep.* **Hyosc. Jod. Ipec.** *Kali.* **Lach.** Laur. **Led.** *Lyc.* **M. arct. Magn. M. mur.** Mang. Mar. Men. Merc. Mezer. Millef. M. ac. Natr. N. mur. *Nitr.* *N. ac.* **N. mosch. N. vom.** Par. **Petr.** *Phosph.* **Ph. ac. Plat.** *Plumb.* Psor. *Puls.* **R. bulb.** *R. scel.* Rheum. Rhod. *Rhus.* Ruta. Sabad. Sabin. **Samb.** *Sassap.* Scill. Selen. **Seneg. Sep. Sil.** Spig.

LEFT SIDE.	RIGHT SIDE.
Veratr. *Verb.* **Viol. od.** Viol. tric. Vit. Zinc.	**Spong.** Stann. Staph. *Sulph. S. ac.* Tar. *Thuj.* Valer. **Veratr.** Verb. Zinc.

NOSE.

Agar. *Amm.* **A. mur.** Anac. A. cr. **Ap.** *Ars.* **Asar.** *Aur. Bell. Bor. Bov.* Brom. **Bry. Calc.** Canth. **Caps.** C. an. **C. veg.** *Caust.* Chel. **Chin. Cina.** Cocc. *Coff. Coloc.* Dros. **Dulc.** Fluor. Graph. **Hell.** Hep. Kali. Laur. Lyc. M. arct. **Magn. M. mur.** Mar. *Merc.* **N. mur.** N. ac. *N. mosch.* **N. vom. Oleand.** Petr. **Phosph.** *Plat.* Psor. Puls. **Rhod. Rhus.** Sabin. **Sassap. Sep.** *Sil.* **Spong.** Stann. *Staph.* **Sulph.** Tar. **Thuj.** V. tr. Zinc.	*Acon.* **Alum. Ambr.** Amm. A. mur. Anac. A. crud. **Asaf. Aur.** *Brom. Bry.* **Calad.** *Calc.* **Canth.** C. an. C. veg. Caust. *Chel.* **Cic.** Cocc. **Colch. Con.** *Croc.* Dros. *Fluor. Graph.* Hep. **Jod.** *Kali.* Laur. *Lyc.* **M. arct. Mang.** *Mar.* Merc. **Natr.** N. mur. **Nitr.** *N. ac.* **N. vom.** Petr. *Phosph. Ph. ac.* Plat. *Psor. Puls. R. bulb.* **R. scel.** *Rhus.* Sabin. Sassap. Sep. *Sil.* **Spig.** Stann. *Sulph.* S. ac. Tar. *Thuj.* **Veratr. V. od.** V. tr. **Vit.** Zinc.

FACE.

Acon. Alum. **Amm.** Anac. **A. cr.** A. tart. **Ap.** Arg. **Arn.** Ars. *Asaf.* **Asar.** Aur. **Bar. Bell. Bor. Bov.** *Brom.* Bry. **Calc.** *Cann.* Canth. *Caps. C. an.* **C. veg. Caust.** Cham. Chel. Chin. *Cic.* **Cina.** *Clem.* Cocc. **Coff.** Colch. *Coloc. Con.* Creos. **Cupr.** *Dig.* Dros. **Dulc. Euph. Euphr.** Fluor. Graph. Guaj. **Hell.** Hep. *Hyosc.* **Ignat.** Jod. Kali. **Lach.** Laur. **Led.** Lyc. **M.** arct. Magn. M. mur.	Acon. **Agar. Alum.** Amm. *A. mur.* **Anac.** A. cr. A. tart. Ap. **Arg.** Arn. *Ars.* Asaf. Asar. *Aur.* **Bar. Bell. Bism.** Bor. Brom. *Bry.* **Calc.** Cann. **Canth.** Caps. C. an. C. veg. *Caust.* Cham. **Chel.** *Chin.* Cina. *Cocc.* **Colch.** Coloc. **Con.** *Creos.* Cupr. **Cycl.** Dig. **Dros. Dulc.** Euphr. *Fluor.* **Graph. Guaj.** *Hep.* Hyosc. Jod. **Kali. Lach.** Laur. Led. **Lyc.** M. arct. **Magn.** M. mur. **Mang. Mar.**

LEFT SIDE.

Mang. Mar. Men. **Merc. Mezer. Millef.** Mosch. *M. ac.* Natr. **N. mur.** Nitr. N. ac. N. mosch. N. vom. *Oleand. Par.* Petr. Phosph. **Ph. ac. Plat.** Plumb. Psor. **Puls.** R. bulb. *Rhod.* **Rhus. Ruta. Sabad. Sabin. Samb. Seneg.**/*Sep.* Sil. Spig. *Spong.* Stann. Staph. Stram. Stront. *Sulph.* S. ac. Tar. **Thuj.** Valer. **Veratr. Verb. V. od.** *V. tr.* Zinc.

RIGHT SIDE.

Men. *Merc.* **Mezer.** Millef. **Mosch.** *Natr.* N. mur. **Nitr.** *N. ac.* **N. mosch. N. vom.** Oleand. Par. Petr. *Phosph.* Ph. ac. Plat. *Plumb. Psor.*/ *Puls.* R. bulb. R. scel. **Rheum.** *Rhus.* Sabad. Sabin. **Sassap. Sep.** *Sil. Spig.* Spong. Stann. *Staph.* Stram. Stront. **Sulph.** S. ac. **Tar. Thuj. Valer.** Veratr. **Verb.** *Vit.* Zinc.

T E E T H.

Acon. *Agar.* **Alum.** Ambr. **Amm. A. mur.** Anac. *Ap. Arn.* **Asaf. Asar. Aur.** *Bar.* Bell. *Bor.* **Brom. Bry. Calc.** Cann. Canth. *C. an. C. veg.* **Caust. Cham. Chel.** *Chin.* **Clem.** Coff. **Colch.** *Con.* **Creos. Croc. Cycl. Euph.** Fluor. Graph. *Guaj.* **Hyosc.** Jod. Kali. *Laur.* **Led.** Lyc. *M. arct.* Mar. *Merc.* **Mezer. Millef.** N. mur. **Nitr.** *N. mosch.* **N. vom. Oleand.** *Phosph.* **Puls.** R. scel. **Rheum.** *Rhod. Rhus.*/Sabad. **Sabin. Samb.** *Selen.* **Seneg. Sep.** *Sil. Spig.* Spong. **Staph.** Stront. **Sulph. Thuj. Veratr.** Verb. *Zinc.*

Agar. Alum. **Ambr. Amm.** Anac. *Ang.* Ap. **Aur.** Bar. **Bell. Bov.** Brom. *Bry. Calc.* **Camph. Cann.** Canth. C. an. C. veg. **Caust. Chin. Coff.** Colch. **Coloc.** Con. *Creos.* **Fluor. Graph.** *Hell. Jod.* Kali. Lach. Laur. Lyc. *Magn.* **Mang. Mar. Merc.** Mezer. **Natr. N. mur. N. ac.** *N. vom.* Oleand. *Petr.* **Ph. ac.** *Psor.* **Puls.** *R. bulb.* R. scel. Rhod. **Rhus. Ruta.** *Sabad.*/*Sassap.* **Sep. Sil.** Spig. Spong. **Staph.** Stront. Sulph. *Tar.* Thuj. **Valer.** *Verb.* **Vit.** Zinc.

MOUTH AND FAUCES.

Acon. Alum. **Ang.** A. crud. **A. tart. Ap. Aur.** Bar. **Bell.** Bov.

Alum. *Amm.* A. crud. **Ars.** Aur. Bov. **Brom. Calc.** *C. veg.*

LEFT SIDE.

Calc. **C. an.** C. veg. *Caust.* **Colch.** Creos. **Croc. Cupr.** Dros. **Euph.** Fluor. *Graph. Hep.* Jod. *Kali. Lach. Lyc.* **M. austr. Mar. Men. Mezer.** Millef. N. mur. **N. ac. N. mosch.** *N. vom.* Oleand. **Phosph.** Ph. ac. Plat. Psor. *Puls.* **Rhod.** *Rhus.* Sabad. **Sabin.** *Seneg.* **Sep. Sil.** Spig. *Sulph.* **Tar. Thuj. Veratr.** *Zinc.*

RIGHT SIDE.

Caust. Chin. Coloc. *Creos. Dros. Fluor.* Graph. Jod. Lach. **M. arct.** Mar. **Merc.** Millef. **N. mur. N. ac. N. vom. Petr.** Plat. **Plumb. Psor. R. bulb.** Rhus. **Sabad. Sep.** Sil. **Spig. Stann. Sulph. Thuj.** Zinc.

HYPOCHONDRIA.

Acon. **Agar.** Alum. Amm. *A. mur.* **Anac.** *A. crud. Ap.* **Arg.** *Arn. Ars.* **Asaf.** *Asar.* **Aur.** Bell. *Bor.*/Brom. **Bry.** Calad. **Calc.** *Cann.* C. an. *C. veg. Caust. Cham.* **Chel.** *Chin.* **Cocc. Coff. Con. Creos.** *Cupr.* **Dig.** Dulc. *Euph. Ferr.* **Fluor. Graph. Hep. Ignat.** Jod. **Ipec. Kali.** Laur. Lyc. Mang. Mar. Merc. *Mezer. Millef.* Mosch. *M. ac.* **Natr. N. mur. Nitr. N. ac. N. vom. Oleand. Par.** Petr. Phosph. Ph. ac. **Plat. Plumb. Puls.** *Psor. R. bulb.* **R. scel.** *Rheum.* **Rhod.** Rhus. **Ruta.** Sabad. **Sassap. Scill. S. corn. Seneg.** *Sep.* **Sil. Spig. Stann. Staph. Sulph. S. ac.** Valer. *Verb.* **V. tric.** *Vit. Zinc.*

Acon. Agar. *Alum. Ambr.* **Amm.** A. mur. *Anac.* **Ang. A. crud.** Ap. **Arn. Ars. Asaf. Bar. Bell.** Bor./**Bry.** Calad. *Calc. Canth. C. an.* **C. veg. Caust.** Chel. **Chin.** *Clem.* **Cocc.** *Colch. Con.* Creos. *Dig.* Dulc. **Ferr.** Fluor. **Graph. Hep. Hyosc. Ignat. Jod. Kali.** *Lach. Laur.* **Led. Lyc. M. arct. M. austr. M. mur.** Mang. **Mar.** *Merc.* Millef. *Mosch.* **Natr.** *N. mur.* N. ac. **N. mosch. N. vom.** Par. *Petr.* Phosph. **Ph. ac.** Plat. **Plumb.** Psor. **Puls. R. bulb. R. scel.** Rhod. **Rhus. Ruta.** *Sabad.* **Sabin.** *S. corn. Selen.* **Sep.** *Sil.* **Spig.** *Stann.* Staph. **Sulph. S. ac.** Valer. *Veratr.* Verb. **Vit.** Zinc.

ABDOMEN.

LEFT SIDE.

Acon. Agar. **Alum.** Ambr. *Amm.* *A. mur.* Anac. Ang. A. crud. *A. tart.* *Ap.* *Arg.* Arn. Ars. **Asaf.** **Asar.** **Aur.** Bar. **Bell.** *Bov.* **Brom.** *Bry.* *Calc.* Camph. **Cann.** Canth. **Caps.** C. veg. Caust. *Cham.* Chel. **Chin.** *Cina.* Cocc. Colch. Coloc. **Con.** **Creos.** Croc. *Cupr.* **Dig.** **Dulc.** **Euph.** **Fluor.** **Graph.** *Guaj.* **Hep.** **Ignat.** **Jod.** *Kali.* Laur. **Led.** Lyc. **M. arct.** M. austr. M. mur. **Mang.** Mar. **Men.** Merc. **Mezer.** *Millef.* **M. ac.** **Natr.** *N. mur.* **N. ac.** N. mosch. **N. vom.** **Oleand.** **Op.** *Par.* Petr. **Ph. ac.** Plat. **Plumb.** **Psor.** *Puls.* *R. bulb.* **Rheum.** Rhod. Rhus. **Ruta.** **Sabad.** Sabin. **Samb.** *Sassap.* Scill. **Selen.** Sep. Sil. *Spig.* **Spong.** Stann. **Staph.** **Sulph.** **S. ac.** **Tar.** Thuj. *Valer.* **Verb.** V. tric. Vit. Zinc.

RIGHT SIDE.

Agar. *Ambr.* A. mur. Anac. **Ang.** **A. crud.** Ap. Arg. **Arn.** **Ars.** Asaf. Aur. *Bar.* Bell. **Bism.** **Bry.** **Calad.** Calc. Camph. Cann. *Canth.* *C. an.* *C. veg.* *Caust.* Chel. Chin. **Cic.** **Clem.** Cocc. **Colch.** *Coloc.* Con. Creos. **Croc.** Cupr. **Cycl.** Dig. **Dros.** Dulc. Fluor. Graph. Guaj. *Ignat.* Jod. **Ipec.** Kali. *Lach.* Laur. *Lyc.* M. austr. *M. mur.* **Mar.** Men. **Merc.** Mezer. Millef. **Mosch.** Natr. N. mur. *Nitr.* N. ac. N. mosch. **N. vom.** Oleand. Petr. **Phosph.** Ph. ac. **Plat.** Plumb. Psor. **Puls.** R. bulb. **R. scel.** Rhod. *Rhus.* Sabad. **Sabin.** Samb. Scill. *Seneg.* *Sep.* Sil. Spig. Spong. *Stann.* **Stront.** Sulph. Tar. *Thuj.* Verb. **V. tric.** **Vit.** Zinc.

ABDOMINAL RINGS.

Agar. **Alum.** **Ambr.** *Amm.* A. mur. **A. crud.** *Ap.* *Arg.* Arn. **Asar.** Aur. Bell. Calc. Camph. Cann. Canth. C. an. **Chel.** Cocc. **Dig.** *Dulc.* **Euph.** Fluor. Graph. *Ignat.* Kali. Laur. Lyc.

Alum. Amm. *A. mur.* **Ap.** **Ars.** *Aur.* **Bell.** **Bor.** **Calc.** Camph. Cann. Canth. C. an. *C. veg.* **Cic.** **Clem.** **Cocc.** *Coloc.* **Con.** Dig. **Dros.** Dulc. Fluor. Graph. **Hell.** **Jod.** **Ipec.** **Kali.** **Lach.** *Laur.*

LEFT SIDE.

M. arct. **M. austr.** **Magn.** **M. mur.** **Merc.** *N. ac.* N. mosch. **N. vom.** **Par.** **Phosph.** Rhod. Rhus. **Sabad.** Sabin. Sassap. **Sep.** Sil. **Spig.** Spong. **Stann.** **Staph.** *Sulph.* **S. ac.** **Tar.** **Veratr.** V. tr. Vit. **Zinc.**

RIGHT SIDE.

Lyc. **Mang.** **Mar.** *Merc.* *Mezer.* **N. vom.** **Op.** *Petr.* **Ph. ac.** **Psor.** **Puls.** **R. bulb.** **Rhod.** **Rhus.** **Ruta.** **Sabin.** Sassap. *Seneg.* **Sep.** *Sil.* Spig. Spong. Stann. *Staph.* *Stront.* Sulph. **S. ac.** **Thuj.** **Valer.** *Veratr.* Vit. Zinc.

SEXUAL ORGANS.

Agar. Alum. Ambr. **A. mur.** *Ang.* **A. cr.** *Ap.* **Arg.** **Aur.** **Bar.** *Brom.* **Bry.** Calc. Cann. **Chin.** Clem. **Colch.** **Con.** **Euph.** *Fluor.* Graph. *Kali.* Lyc. M. arct. *Magn.* Mar. Men. **Merc.** Mezer. **Natr.** *N. ac.* Petr. *Ph. ac.* **Plumb.** **Puls.** *Rhod.* **Rhus.** **Sabad.** Selen. **Sep.** Sil. Spig. Staph. Tar. **Thuj.** Zinc.

Acon. Alum. **Ap.** *Arn.* *Aur.* **Bism.** **Calc.** **Cann.** **Canth.** **Caust.** *Clem.* **Coff.** *Coloc.* *Con.* **Croc.** Graph. **Hep.** *Jod.* *Lach.* *Lyc.* M. arct. Mar. *Men.* *Merc.* Mezer. **M. ac.** N. ac. **N. vom.** Petr. *Puls.* **Rhod.** *Sabin.* **S. corn.** **Selen.** Sil. *Spig.* **Spong.** *Staph.* *Sulph.* **S. ac.** Tar. **Valer.** **Veratr.** *Zinc.*

NECK AND NAPE OF THE NECK.

Acon. Alum. **A. mur.** **Anac.** Ang. **Ap.** **A. crud.** Arg. **Arn.** Ars. **Asaf.** *Asar.* Aur. **Bar.** Bell. **Bor.** **Bov.** **Brom.** **Bry.** **Calc.** **Canth.** **C. an.** **C. veg.** Caust. **Cic.** Cocc. Colch. **Coloc.** **Croc.** **Cycl.** Fluor. *Guaj.* **Hyosc.** **Ignat.** Kali. Lach. Laur. *Lyc.* Mar. Merc. Mezer. **Mosch.** **N. vom.** *Oleand.* **Par.** Ph. ac. **Psor.** Rhod. **Rhus.** *Sabin.* **Scil.** *Selen.* **Sep.** **Sil.** Spig. **Spong.**

Alum. **Amm.** Anac. Ang. A. cr. **A. tart.** Ap. **Arg.** Asaf. Aur. *Bell.* *Bism.* Bry. **Calc.** **Camph.** Canth. **Caps.** C. veg. **Caust.** **Chel.** **Chin.** **Cina.** Cocc. *Colch.* Coloc. *Con.* **Cupr.** **Dulc.** **Fluor.** Guaj. *Hep.* *Jod.* *Kali.* *Lach.* *Laur.* **Led.** **Lyc.** **M. austr.** **Mar.** **Men.** **Merc.** *Mezer.* **Natr.** **N. mur.** **Nitr.** **N. ac.** *N. vom.* Oleand. **Petr.** Ph. ac. **Plat.** **Plumb.** **Puls.** Rhod. Sabin. *Sas-*

LEFT SIDE.

Staph. *Stram.* **Sulph.** **S. ac.** *Tar.* *Thuj.* **Veratr.** **V. tr.** Vit. Zinc.

RIGHT SIDE.

sap. Seneg. Sil. **Spig.** *Spong.* **Staph.** **Sulph.** *S. ac.* Thuj. Vit. Zinc.

CHEST.

Acon. **Agar.** Alum. Ambr. **Amm.** **A. mur.** **Anac.** Ang. **A. cr.** *A. tart.* *Ap.* Arg. *Arn.* Ars. **Asaf.** Asar. **Aur.** **Bar.** **Bell.** **Bism.** Bor. **Bov.** Brom. **Bry.** **Calad.** **Calc.** **Camph.** *Cann.* **Canth.** *Caps.* **C. an.** *C. veg.* *Caust.* *Cham.* **Chel.** *Chin.* Cic. *Cina.* Clem. *Cocc.* Colch. Coloc. **Con.** *Creos.* **Croc.** **Cupr.** **Cycl.** Dig. **Dros.** *Dulc.* **Euph.** **Fluor.** *Graph.* *Guaj.* **Hep.** Hyosc. *Ignat.* **Kali.** Lach. **Laur.** Led. **Lyc.** Mgs. *M. arct.* *M. austr.* **Magn.** Mang. Mar. *Men.* *Merc.* Mezer. Millef. **Mosch.** M. ac. **Natr.** *N. mur.* *Nitr.* **N. ac.** N. mosch. **N. vom.** *Oleand.* Par. Petr. *Phosph.* *Ph. ac.* **Plat.** *Plumb.* Psor. **Puls.** *R. bulb.* R. scel. **Rheum.** *Rhod.* **Rhus.** *Ruta.* Sabad. *Sabin.* Sassap. **Scill.** **Seneg.** *Sep.* **Sil.** *Spig.* *Spong.* **Stann.** **Staph.** Stront. **Sulph.** *S. ac.* **Tar.** *Thuj.* *Valer.* **Veratr.** *Verb.* *V. tr.* Vit. *Zinc.*

Acon. Agar. **Alum.** Ambr. *Amm.* A. mur. Anac. Ang. A. cr. A. tart. **Arg.** **Arn.** **Ars.** *Asaf.* Asar. *Aur.* Bar. **Bell.** Bism. *Bor.* Bov. *Brom.* **Bry.** Calad. **Calc.** Camph. **Cann.** *Canth.* Caps. **C. an.** **C. veg.** Caust. **Cham.** Chel. Chin. Cic. Cina. Clem. **Cocc.** *Colch.* **Coloc.** Con. Creos. Croc. Cupr. Cycl. *Dig.* Dros. **Dulc.** Euph. Fluor. **Graph.** *Hep.* *Hyosc.* Ignat. **Jod.** **Ipec.** Kali. **Lach.** Laur. *Led.* **Lyc.** *Mgs.* **M. arct.** M. austr. *M. mur.* Mang. **Mar.** Men. **Merc.** Mezer. Millef. *M. ac.* Natr. **N. mur.** Nitr. **N. ac.** **N. mosch.** **N. vom.** Oleand. *Op.* **Par.** Petr. *Phosph.* **Ph. ac.** Plat. Plumb. **Psor.** **Puls.** **R. bulb.** **R. scel.** Rheum. **Rhus.** Ruta. **Sabad.** Sabin. Sassap. *Scill.* Seneg. **Sep.** **Sil.** **Spig.** Spong. Stann. Staph. Stront. **Sulph.** S. ac. *Tar.* Thuj. Valer. *Veratr.* **V. tric.** **Vit.** Zinc.

BACK.

Acon. *Agar.* *Alum.* Ambr. **Amm.** A. mur. *Anac.* Ang. A. cr. A. tart.

Acon. Agar. Alum. Ambr. Amm. **A. mur.** Anac. Ang. **A. cr.** **A.**

LEFT SIDE.

Ap. Arg. **Ars.** **Asaf.** Aur. *Bar.* Bell. *Bism.* *Bry.* Calc. Cann. Canth. C. an. **C. veg.** *Caust.* Chel. *Chin.* Cina. **Cocc.** Colch. **Coloc.** Con. **Creos.** **Croc.** **Cupr.** **Dig.** **Dros.** **Dulc.** Euph. **Ferr.** **Fluor.** *Graph.* Guaj. **Hell.** *Hep.* *Ignat.* Jod. *Kali.* Laur. **Led.** **Lyc.** **Mgs.** **M. austr.** *Mang.* *Mar.* Men. Merc. Mezer. **Millef.** **Mosch.** M. ac. **N. mur.** **Nitr.** N. ac. N. vom. Oleand. *Par.* **Petr.** Phosph. **Ph. ac.** Plat. Plumb. **Psor.** *Puls.* R. scel. **Rhod.** **Rhus.** *Ruta.* Sabad. *Sabin.* Sassap. *Scill.* *Seneg.* Sep. **Sil.** **Spig.** *Spong.* *Stann.* **Staph.** **Stront.** *Sulph.* S. ac. Tar. **Thuj.** *Valer.* *Veratr.* Verb. V. tric. Vit. Zinc.

RIGHT SIDE.

tart. Ap. **Arg.** *Arn.* *Ars.* Asaf. **Asar.** **Aur.** Bar. Bell. **Bor.** **Brom.** **Bry.** **Calc.** Cann. *Canth.* *C. an.* C. veg. **Caust.** Chel. **Chin.** **Cic.** Cina. Cocc. **Colch.** *Coloc.* *Con.* Cupr. Dig. Dros. Dulc. *Euph.* **Fluor.** *Guaj.* Hep. **Jod.** **Kali.** *Laur.* *Lyc.* *M. arct.* M. austr. Mar. Men. Merc. Mezer. Millef. Mur. ac. *N. mur.* N. ac. *N. vom.* *Oleand.* Petr. *Phosph.* Plat. **Plumb.** *R. bulb.* R. scel. Rhod. *Rhus.* Ruta. **Sabad.** *Samb.* Sassap. **Sep.** **Sil.** Spig. Spong. Stann. Staph. **Sulph.** S. ac. *Tar.* Thuj. Verb. V. tric. Vit. **Zinc.**

UPPER EXTREMITIES.

Acon. Agar. *Alum.* Ambr. Amm. A. mur. **Anac.** Ang. A. crud. **A. tart.** *Ap.* Arg. **Arn.** **Ars.** **Asaf.** Asar. Aur. *Bar.* **Bell.** Bism. Bor. Bov. **Brom.** **Bry.** **Calad.** **Calc.** **Camph.** Cann. Canth. *Caps.* C. an. **C. veg.** Caust. *Cham.* Chel. **Chin.** **Cic.** **Cina.** Clem. **Cocc.** **Coff.** Colch. Coloc. **Con.** *Creos.* **Croc.** Cupr. **Cycl.** Dig. Dros. Dulc. Euph. *Euphr.* Ferr. *Fluor.* Graph. Guaj. Hell. *Hep.* **Hyosc.** **Ignat.** **Jod.**

Acon. Agar. Alum. *Ambr.* Amm. **A. mur.** Anac. *Ang.* **A. crud.** A. tart. **Ap.** Arg. Arn. *Ars.* Asaf. Asar. *Aur.* Bar. **Bell.** **Bism.** *Bor.* *Bov.* Brom. **Bry.** Calad. **Calc.** Camph. *Cann.* *Canth.* Caps. C. an. **C. veg.** **Caust.** **Cham.** **Chel.** Chin. Cic. Cina. Clem. *Cocc.* Coff. *Colch.* **Coloc.** **Con.** Creos. Croc. *Cupr.* Cycl. **Dig.** **Dros.** **Dulc.** Euph. Euphr. **Ferr.** Fluor. **Graph.** Guaj. Hell. Hep. Hyosc. *Ignat.* Jod.

LEFT SIDE.

Ipec. **Kali.** **Lach.** Laur. **Led.** *Lyc.* Mgs. *M. arct.* **M. austr.** Magn. *M. mur.* Mang. *Mar.* **Men.** **Merc.** Mezer. Millef. **Mosch.** **M. ac.** Natr. **N. mur.** **Nitr.** **N. ac.** **N. mosch.** **N. vom.** *Oleand.* **Op.** Par. *Petr.* Phosph. *Ph. ac.* Plat. Plumb. **Psor.** **Puls.** R. bulb. R. scel. Rheum. Rhod. **Rhus.** Ruta. Sabad. **Sabin.** Samb. Sassap. **Scill.** S. corn. **Selen.** *Seneg.* **Sep.** **Sil.** Spig. Spong. **Stann.** **Staph.** **Stram.** **Stront.** **Sulph.** S. ac. *Tar.* **Thuj.** *Valer.* **Veratr.** *Verb.* Viol. od. *V. tric.* Vit. **Zinc.**

RIGHT SIDE.

Ipec. Kali. *Lach.* Laur. Led. **Lyc.** **Mgs.** M. arct. M. austr. **Magn.** M. mur. *Mang.* Mar. Men. Merc. Mezer. Millef. Mosch. M. ac. *Natr.* N. mur. Nitr. N. ac. N. mosch. *N. vom.* Oleand. Op. Par. **Petr.** **Phosph.** **Ph. ac.** Plat. *Plumb.* *Psor.* **Puls.** R. bulb. R. scel. **Rheum.** **Rhod.** **Rhus.** Ruta. Sabad. Sabin. Samb. **Sassap.** Scill. S. corn. Selen. Seneg. **Sep.** **Sil.** Spig. Spong. Stann. **Staph.** Stram. Stront. **Sulph.** *S. ac.* Tar. **Thuj.** Valer. Veratr. Verb. **Viol. od.** V. tr. **Vit.** **Zinc.**

LOWER EXTREMITIES.

Acon. *Agar.* Alum. **Ambr.** **Amm.** **A. mur.** **Anac.** Ang. A. crud. *A. tart.* *Ap.* *Arg.* Arn. **Ars.** **Asaf.** **Asar.** Aur. **Bar.** **Bell.** Bism. **Bor.** **Bov.** Brom. **Bry.** *Calad.* **Calc.** Camph. Cann. Canth. Caps. C. an. **C. veg.** *Caust.* Cham. **Chel.** Chin. *Cic.* **Cina.** **Clem.** **Cocc.** Coff. Colch. **Coloc.** **Con.** *Creos.* *Croc.* Cupr. Cycl. **Dig.** Dros. **Dulc.** **Euph.** **Euphr.** **Ferr.** **Fluor.** **Graph.** **Guaj.** *Hell.* **Hep.** *Hyosc.* **Ignat.** *Jod.* Ipec. Kali. **Lach.** Laur. **Led.** **Lyc.** **Mgs.** M. arct. *M. austr.* *Magn.* M. mur. Mang. **Mar.** Men.

Acon. Agar. **Alum.** Ambr. Amm. A. mur. Anac. **Ang.** A. crud. A. tart. **Ap.** **Arg.** *Arn.* **Ars.** Asaf. Asar. *Aur.* Bar. **Bell.** Bism. Bor. Bov. **Brom.** **Bry.** Calad. **Calc.** **Camph.** Cann. *Canth.* Cap. **C. an.** **C. veg.** **Caust.** Cham. Chel. **Chin.** Cic. Cina. Clem. *Cocc.* *Coff.* Colch. **Coloc.** *Con.* Creos. Croc. **Cupr.** Cycl. Dig. **Dros.** Dulc. Euph. Euphr. Ferr. *Fluor.* **Graph.** **Guaj.** Hell. **Hep.** Hyosc. **Ignat.** Jod. Ipec. Kali. **Lach.** *Laur.* **Led.** **Lyc.** Mgs. M. arct. M. austr. *Magn.* M. mur. Mang.

LEFT SIDE.

Merc. *Mezer.* Millef. **Mosch.** M. ac. Natr. N. mur. Nitr. **N. ac.** N. mosch. **N. vom.** Oleand. Op. Par. **Petr.** **Phosph.** Ph. ac. **Plat.** Plumb. **Psor.** **Puls.** **R. bulb.** R. scel. *Rheum.* Rhod. **Rhus.** *Ruta.* Sabad. *Sabin.* Samb. Sassap. Scill. S. corn. *Selen.* **Seneg.** **Sep.** **Sil.** **Spig.** Spong. **Stann.** Staph. Stram. **Stront.** **Sulph.** *S. ac.* Tar. Thuj. **Valer.** **Verat.** Verb. V. od. V. tr. **Vit.** *Zinc.*

RIGHT SIDE.

Mar. **Men.** **Merc.** **Mezer.** **Millef.** Mosch. M. ac. **Natr.** **N. mur.** **Nitr.** **N. ac.** *N. mosch.* **N. vom.** **Oleand.** Op. *Par.* **Petr.** **Phosph.** *Ph. ac.* Plat. Plumb. **Psor.** **Puls.** R. bulb. *R. scel.* Rheum. **Rhod.** **Rhus.** Ruta. *Sabad.* **Sabin.** *Samb.* **Sassap.** Scill. **S. corn.** Selen. Seneg. **Sep.** **Sil.** Spig. **Spong.** Stann. *Staph.* **Stram.** Stront. **Sulph.** S. ac. *Tar.* *Thuj.* Valer. *Veratr.* *Verb.* V. od. *V. tr.* Vit. **Zinc.**

GENERAL SYMPTOMS.

Acon. **Agar.** Alum. Ambr. Amm. A. mur. *Anac.* Ang. *A. crud.* *A. tart.* **Ap.** **Arg.** **Arn.** Ars. **Asaf.** **Asar.** Aur. **Bar.** Bell. Bism. Bor. **Bov.** *Brom.* Bry. Calad. Calc. Camph. Cann. Canth. **Caps.** C. an. C. veg. Caust. *Cham.* Chel. *Chin.* Cic. **Cina.** **Clem.** Cocc. Coff. Colch. Coloc. Con. *Creos.* **Croc.** **Cupr.** Cycl. **Dig.** Dros. *Dulc.* **Euph.** *Euphr.* *Ferr.* Fluor. Graph. *Guaj.* Hell. Hep. Hyosc. **Ignat.** Jod. Ipec. Kali. Lach. Laur. Led. Lyc. Mgs. *M. arct.* **M. austr.** **Magn.** M. mur. Mang. Mar. Men. Merc. **Mezer.** **Millef.** Mosch. *M. ac.* Natr. N. mur. Nitr. **N. ac.** N. mosch. N. vom. **Oleand.** Op. *Par.*

Acon. Agar. **Alum.** Ambr. Amm. A. mur. Anac. **Ang.** A. cr. A. tart. Ap. Arg. Arn. Ars. Asaf. Asar. **Aur.** Bar. **Bell.** *Bism.* Bor. Bov. Brom. *Bry.* Calad. **Calc.** Camph. **Cann.** **Canth.** Caps. C. an. C. veg. **Caust.** Cham. Chel. Chin. Cic. Cina. Clem. **Cocc.** Coff. *Colch.* **Coloc.** *Con.* Creos. Croc. Cupr. Cycl. Dig. **Dros.** Dulc. Euph. Euphr. Ferr. **Fluor.** Graph. Guaj. Hell. Hep. Hyosc. Ignat. *Jod.* *Ipec.* Kali. **Lach.** Laur. Led. **Lyc.** **Mgs.** M. arct. M. austr. Magn. *M. mur.* *Mang.* *Mar.* Men. Merc. Mezer. Millef. **Mosch.** M. ac. *Natr.* N. mur. **Nitr.** N. ac. *N. mosch.* **N. vom.** Oleand. **Op.** Par. *Petr.*

LEFT SIDE.	RIGHT SIDE.
Petr. Phosph. Ph. ac. Plat. Plumb. Psor. Puls. R. bulb. R. scel. *Rheum.* Rhod. Rhus. *Ruta.* Sabad. *Sabin.* Samb. Sassap. **Scill.** S. corn. **Selen.** Seneg. Sep. Sil. *Spig.* Spong. **Stann.** Staph. **Stram.** Stront. **Sulph.** S. ac. **Tar.** **Thuj.** **Valer.** Veratr. **Verb.** *V. odor.* *V. tric.* Vit. **Zinc.**	**Phosph.** Ph. ac. Plat. **Plumb.** Psor. *Puls.* *R. bulb.* **R. scel.** Rheum. Rhod. *Rhus.* Ruta. *Sabad.* Sabin. Samb. **Sassap.** Scill. **S. corn.** Selen. Seneg. Sep. *Sil.* Spig. Spong. Stann. *Staph.* Stram. **Stront.** Sulph. **S. ac.** Tar. Thuj. Valer. **Veratr.** Verb. **Viol.** od. Viol. tric. *Vit.* Zinc.

CROSS-WISE.

LEFT UPPER SIDE. RIGHT LOWER SIDE.	LEFT LOWER SIDE. RIGHT UPPER SIDE.
Alum. *Anac.* *Arn.* Ars. **Bar.** **Bell.** **Brom.** Camph. Caps. *C. an.* Cham. **Chin.** **Coff.** **Con.** Cycl. Euphr. *Fluor.* Hep. *Kali.* Lach. Laur. Led. M. arct. M. austr. M. mur. **Mar.** Men. **Merc.** Millef. M. ac. N. mur. Nitr. N. ac. **N. mosch.** N. vom. **Oleand.** Op. **Par.** **Ph. ac.** *Puls.* R. scel. Rhod. *Rhus.* Sabad. **Sabin.** Samb. **Sassap.** *Scill.* **S. corn.** **Seneg.** Spong. *Stann.* **Staph.** Stram. **Sulph.** **Tar.** *Thuj.* Valer. *Veratr.* *Verb.* *V. tric.*	**Acon.** **Agar.** **Ambr.** Amm. A. mur. Ang. A. crud. A. tart. **Arg.** Asar. **Bism.** *Bor.* *Bov.* Bry. Calad. *Calc.* Cann. C. veg. *Caust.* Chel. Cic. **Cina.** Colch. **Coloc.** Croc. Cupr. **Dig.** Dulc. Euph. **Euphr.** *Ferr.* Graph. Hell. Hyosc. Ignat. Jod. Ipec. *Lyc.* Mgs. Magn. Mang. Mezer. **M. ac.** Natr. **N. vom.** **Phosph.** Plat. *Plumb.* R. bulb. **Rheum.** **Rhus.** Ruta. Selen. *Sil.* Spig. **S. ac.** V. od. Vit.

FEBRILE SYMPTOMS.

Agar. Ambr. **A. crud.** Arn. **Bar.** Caust. Cham. *Chin.* Dig. **Lyc.** **Par.** *Plat.* Puls. **Rhus.** Ruta. **Spig.** **Stann.** **Sulph.** **Thuj.** **Verb.** **Vit.**	Ambr. *Bell.* **Bry.** **Caust.** Chin. Cocc. **Fluor.** Natr. *N. vom.* **Phosph.** **Puls.** *R. bulb.* **Sabin.** Spig. Verb.

DRUG-AFFINITIES.

ACON.—*Arn.* *Ars.* **Bell.** **Bry.** **Canth.** **Cham.** *Coff.* **Croc.** **Dulc.** **Graph.** *Lyc.* **Merc.** *Millef.* *N. vom.* *Op.* *Phosph.* *Ph. ac.* *Puls.* **Rhus.** **Ruta.** **Sep.** *Sulph.* *Valer.* **Veratr.**

AGAR.—*Bell.* **Calc.** *Cocc.* **Coff.** **Lyc.** *N. ac.* **N. vom.** *Petr.* *Phosph.* *Puls.* *Sep.* **Sil.** *Sulph.*

ALUM.—**Bry.** *Calc.* *Cham.* **Ignat.** *Ipec.* **Lach.** *Lyc.* *N. mur.* **Phosph.** **Plumb.** *Puls.* **Veratr.**

AMBR.—*Bell.* *Calc.* *Lyc.* *N. vom.* *Puls.* **Staph.** *Sulph.*

AMM.—*Brom.* *Calc.* **Fluor.** *Hep.* *Phosph.* *S. corn.*

A. MUR.—*Ars.* **N. vom.** *Puls.* *Rhus.*

ANAC.—**Calc.** *Coff.* *Con.* *N. mur.*

ANG.—**Bry.** **Calc.** **Lyc.** *Rhus.* **Verb.**

A. CRUD.—*Ars.* **Bism.** **Brom.** **Hep.** **Ipec.** **Merc.** **Puls.** *Sep.* **Sulph.**

A. TART.—**Bell.** *Chin.* *Coc.* **Con.** *Ipec.* *Op.* *Puls.* *Sep.*

APIS M.—**Ars.** *Bell.* *Canth.* *Chin.* **Ferr.** **Graph.** **Hep.** **Jod.** **Kali.** **Lach.** *Lyc.* **Merc.** **Millef.** **Puls.** Sep. *Sulph.*

ARG.—**Merc.**

ARN.—*Acon.* *Ars.* **Bry.** **Cann.** **Caps.** *Chin.* **Cic.** *Ferr.* *Ignat.* **Ipec.** **Merc.** **Millef.** *Puls.* **Rhus.** **Sabin.** **Samb.** *Scill.* *Seneg.* *Veratr.* **Zinc.**

ARS.—**Acon.** **A. mur.** *Ant. cr.* *Arn.* **Ap.** *Bar.* **Brom.** *Bry.* **Calc.** *C. veg.* **Cham.** **Chin.** **Coff.** *Dig.* **Colch.** **Dulc.** **Euph.** **Ferr.** *Graph.* **Hep.** *Ignat.* **Jod.** **Ipec.** **Kali.** *Lach.* **Lyc.** **Magn.** **Merc.**

Mosch. **M. ac.** *N. mur.* **N. vom.** *Petr.* *Phosph.* *Ph. ac.* **Plumb.** **R. scel.** *Samb.* *Scill.* *S. corn.* *Sep.* *Sil.* **Stann.** *Staph.* **Sulph.** **S. ac.** *Veratr.*

ASAF.—**Aur.** *Caust.* **Chin.** **Men.** **Merc.** *N. ac.* *Ph. ac.* **Plat.** *Puls.* *Sep.*

ASAR.—**Cupr.** **N. vom.** **Phosph.**

AUR.—**Asaf.** **Calc.** **Coff.** *Merc.* *N. vom.* *Puls.* **Phosph.**

BAR.—*Ars.* **Calc.** **N. vom.** **Sep.** **Zinc.**

BELL.—**Acon.** *Agar.* *Ambr.* *A. tart.* *Ap.* *Bry.* **Calc.** *Cann.* *Canth.* *Caust.* *Cham.* *Chin.* **Cic.** **Cina.** *Coff.* *Colch.* *Coloc.* *Croc.* *Cupr.* **Dig.** *Graph.* **Hell.** **Hep.** **Hyosc.** *Jod.* **Lach.** *Merc.* **Mosch.** *N. ac.* **N. vom.** *Op.* *Ph. ac.* **Plat.** *Plumb.* **Puls.** *Rheum.* *Rhus.* *Sassap.* *Seneg.* **Sep.** **Sil.** *Stram.* **Sulph.** *Valer.*

BISM.—**A. crud.** **Calc.** **Cocc.** **Ignat.** **Spig.** **Staph.**

BOR.—Bry. *Calc.* *Cham.* **Coff.** *Sil.* Sulph.

BOV.—**N. ac.** *Selen.* **Sil.**

BROM.—**Amm.** **A. crud.** **Ars.** **Camph.** **Coff.** *Hep.* *Jod.* **Magn.** **N. mur.** **Op.** **Phosph.** *Spong.*

BRY.—**Acon.** **Alum.** **Ang.** *Ars.* **Bell.** **Bor.** *Calc.* *C. veg.* **Caust.** *Chin.* *Clem.* **Coloc.** *Dulc.* **Guaj.** *Jod.* Ipec. *Kali.* *Led.* *Lyc.* *Mezer.* **Millef.** **Phosph.** *R. bulb.* **Puls.** **Rhod.** **Rhus.** **Scill.** *Seneg.* **Sep.** **Veratr.**

CALAD.—**Canth.** **Caps.** **Ignat.** **N. vom.**

CALC.—**Agar.** **Alum.** *Ambr.* *Amm.* **Anac.** **Ang.** **Ars.** **Aur.** **Bar.** **Bell.** **Bism.** *Bor.* *Bry.* *Cann.* **Caust.** **Chel.** *Chin.* *Cocc.* **Cupr.** *Fluor.* **Graph.** **Ignat.** **Jod.** **Ipec.** *Kali.* **Lyc.** *M. mur.* **Men.** **Merc.** **Natr.** **Nitr.** **N. ac.** **N. vom.** *Petr.* *Phosph.* *Ph. ac.* **Puls.** *Rhus.* **Sabin.** **Sassap.** *Selen.* *Sep.* **Sil.** **Sulph.** **Veratr.** **Vit.**

CAMPH.—**Brom.** *Canth.* **Op.** **Veratr.**

CANN.—**Arn.** *Bell.* *Calc.* **Canth.** **Coloc.** *Euph.* Men. **N. mur.** *N. ac.* *Puls.* *Thuj.*

CANTH.—**Acon.** *Ap.* *Bell.* **Calad.** *Camph.* **Cann.** *Laur.* **Lyc.** **Puls.**

CAPS.—**Arn. Calad. Cham. Chin. Cina. Ignat. N. vom. Puls.**

C. AN.—**C. veg. Rhod. Thuj.**

C. VEG.—*Ars. Bry.* **C. an. Chin. Dulc.** *Ferr. Ignat.* **Ipec. Kali.** *Lach.* **Merc.** *N. mur.* **N. ac.** *N. vom.* **Op.** *Petr. Puls.* **Rhod. Sep.** *Sulph.* **Veratr.**

CAUST.—*Asaf. Bell. Bry.* **Calc. Cocc.** *Clem.* **Coloc. Creos.** *Cupr. Graph.* **Hep.** *Ignat.* **Lach. Lyc. Natr.** *N. vom. Phosph. Plat. Puls. Rhod. Rhus.* **Sep.** *Sil.* **Sulph.**

CHAM.—**Acon. Alum.** *Ars. Bell. Bor.* **Caps.** *Chin. Cina.* **Cocc.** *Coff.* **Coloc. Hep. Ignat. Ipec. Lyc. Magn. N. vom. Petr. Puls.** *Rheum.* **Rhus. Stram.** *Sulph. Valer.*

CHEL.—**Calc. Lyc. Puls. Sulph.**

CHIN.—**Amm.** *A. tart. Ap.* **Arn. Ars. Asaf. Bell.** *Bry. Calc.* **Caps. C. veg.** *Cham. Cina. Cupr.* **Cicl. Dig. Ferr. Fluor.** *Hell. Jod.* **Ipec. Lach. Merc. Millef.** *N. mur.* **N. vom. Phosph.** *Ph. ac.* **Plumb. Puls. Samb.** *Sep.* **Stann.** *Sulph.* **S. ac. Veratr.**

CIC.—**Arn. Bell. Dulc. Lyc. Merc. Op. Rhus. Stram. Veratr.**

CINA.—**Bell. Caps.** *Chin.* **Dros. Hyosc. Merc. Phosph. Veratr.**

CLEM.—*Bry. Graph. Merc.* **Rhod.** *Rhus.*

COCC.—**Agar.** *A. tart.* **Bism.** *Calc.* **Caust. Cham.** *Cupr.* **Ignat. Ipec. Kali. Mosch. N. mosch.** *N. vom.* **Oleand.**

COFF.—*Acon.* **Agar. Anac. Ars. Aur.** *Bell.* **Bor. Brom. Caps.** *Cham.* **Coloc. Con.** *Ignat.* **Magn. Mar. Merc. Mosch.** *N. vom. Op. Puls.* **Sulph.** *Valer. Veratr.*

COLCH.—**Ars.** *Bell. Fluor.* **Merc.** *N. vom.* **Op.** *Puls.*

COLOC.—*Bell.* **Bry. Cann.** *Caust.* **Cham. Coff. Magn.** *Rheum. S. corn.* **Staph.**

CON.—**Anac. A. tart. Coff. Cupr. Cycl. Dig. Dulc. Lach.** *Lyc. N. ac.* **N. vom.** *Puls.* **Vit.**

CREOS.—**Caust.** *N. mur.* **N. vom.** *Sep. Sulph.*

CROC.—**Acon. Bell.** *Op.* **Plat.**

CUPR.—*Bell.* **Calc.** *Caust. Chin. Cocc.* **Con.** *Dulc.* **Hep.** *Hyosc. Ignat. Ipec. Lyc. Merc. N. vom. Op.* **Ph. ac. Puls. Sep. Sil. Sulph. Veratr.**

CYCL.—**Con.** *Puls.*

DIG.—*Ars.* **Bell. Chin. Con. Merc.** *N. vom. Op.* **Phosph. Ph. ac.** *Plat. Puls.* **Spig. S. ac.**

DROS.—**Cina. Hep.** *Ipec.* **N. vom. Sep.** *Spong. Veratr.*

DULC.—**Acon. Ars.** *Bry.* **Cic. Con.** *Cupr.* **Led.** *Merc.* **N. vom. Ph. ac. Puls.** *Rhus. Sep.* **Sulph.**

EUPH.—**Ars. Lyc.** *Merc.* **Mezer.** *Puls.* **Rhus. Sep.** *Zinc.*

EUPHR.—*Cann. Hep. N. vom.* **Spig.**

FERR.—**Ap.** *Arn.* **Ars.** *C. veg. Chin.* **Hep.** *Ipec. Puls. Sulph.* **S. ac.** *Veratr.*

FLUOR.—**Amm.** *Calc.* **Chin.** *Colch.* **Graph. N. ac.** *Sil.*

GRAPH.—**Acon. Ap.** *Ars. Bell.* Calc. *Caust.* **Fluor. Guaj. Kali.** *Lyc.* **Magn. Natr. N. ac.** *N. vom. Phosph.* **Puls.** *Sep.* **Sil. Sulph.** *Thuj.* **Vit.**

GUAJ.—**Bry. Graph. Merc.**

HELL.—**Bell.** *Chin.* **Phosph.**

HEP.—*Amm.* **A. crud. Ap. Ars. Bell.** *Brom.* **Caust. Cham. Cupr. Dros.** *Euphr.* **Ferr. Ignat. Jod. Lach. Lyc. Merc.** *N. ac. Rhus. Sep.* **Sil. Spong. Sulph.** *Thuj.* **Zinc.**

HYOSC.—**Bell.** *Cina. Cupr.* **Op.** *Ph. ac. Plumb.* **Stram.** *Valer. Veratr.*

IGNAT.—**Alum.** *Arn. Ars. Bism.* **Calad. Calc. Caps.** *C. veg. Caust.* **Cham. Cocc.** *Coff. Cupr.* **Hep. Ipec. Lyc. Mar.** *Mgs. M. arct. M. austr. N. vom.* **Ph. ac.** *Plat. Puls.* **Ruta.** *Selen.* **Stram. Valer. Zinc.**

JOD.—**Ap. Ars.** *Bell. Brom. Bry.* **Calc.** *Chin.* **Hep. Kali. Lyc.** *Merc. Par. Phosph.* **Sil.** *Spong.* **Sulph.**

IPEC.—*Alum.* **A. crud.** **A. tart.** **Arn.** **Ars.** **Bry.** **Calc.** **C. veg.** **Cham.** *Chin.* **Cocc.** *Cupr.* *Dros.* *Ferr.* **Ignat.** *Laur.* *Nitr.* **N. vom.** **Op.** **Phosph.** *Puls.* **S. ac.** *Veratr.*

KALI.—**Ap.** *Ars.* *Bry.* *Calc.* **C. veg.** **Cocc.** **Laur.** *Lyc.* *Magn.* *Natr.* *N. mur.* **N. ac.** **N. vom.** *Phosph.* **Puls.** **Sil.**

LACH.—**Alum.** **Ap.** *Ars.* **Bell.** **C. veg.** **Caust.** **Chin.** **Con.** **Hep.** **Lyc.** **Merc.** *N. vom.* *Ph. ac.* **Plat.** **Puls.** *Stann.* **Zinc.**

LAUR.—*Canth.* *Ipec.* **Kali.** **Merc.** **Spig.**

LED.—*Bry.* **Dulc.** **Lyc.** **Puls.**

LYC.—**Acon.** *Agar.* **Alum.** **Ambr.** **Ang.** *Ap.* **Ars.** *Bry.* **Calc.** **Canth.** **Caust.** **Cham.** **Chel.** **Chin.** **Cic.** *Con.* *Cupr.* **Euph.** *Graph.* **Hep.** **Ignat.** **Jod.** *Kali.* **Lach.** **Led.** **M. mur.** *Mang.* **Merc.** *M. ac.* **Natr.** N. ac. **N. vom.** *Petr.* **Phosph.** **Ph. ac.** **Puls.** *Rhus.* *Sep.* **Sil.** **Vit.**

MGS.—*Ignat.* **Zinc.**

M. ARCT.—**Bell.** *Ignat.* *M. austr.* *Puls.* *Zinc.*

M. AUSTR.—*Ignat.* *M. arct.* *N. vom.* *Zinc.*

MAGN.—*Ars.* **Brom.** *Cham.* **Coff.** *Coloc.* **Graph.** *Kali.* **M. mur.** *N. vom.* *Puls.* *Rheum.*

M. MUR.—*Calc.* **Lyc.** **Magn.** **N. vom.** **Sep.** **Sulph.**

MANG.—**Bry.** *Lyc.* **Puls.**

MAR.—**Coff.** **Ignat.**

MEN.—**Asaf.** **Calc.** **Cann.** **Plat.** **Sep.**

MERC.—**Acon.** **A. crud.** **Ap.** **Arg.** **Arn.** **Ars.** **Asaf.** *Aur.* **Bell.** **Bry.** *Calc.* **C. veg.** **Chin.** **Cic.** **Cina.** **Clem.** **Coff.** **Colch.** *Cupr.* **Dig.** *Dulc.* **Euph.** **Guaj.** **Hep.** *Jod.* **Lach.** **Laur.** **Lyc.** *Mezer.* **N. ac.** **N. vom.** **Op.** **Ph. ac.** **Plat.** *Puls.* **Rheum.** **Rhod.** **Rhus.** *Sassap.* **Selen.** **Sep.** *Sil.* *Spig.* **Staph.** **Sulph.** *Thuj.* **Valer.** **Veratr.** **Vit.** *Zinc.*

MEZER.—*Bry.* **Euph.** *Merc.* **M. ac.** *N. ac.* *Rhus.* **Sil.** **Verb.**

MILLEF.—*Acon.* **Ap.** **Arn.** **Bry.** **Chin.** **N. vom.** **Puls.** *Scill.*

MOSCH.—**Bell.** **Cocc.** **Coff.** **N. vom.** **Op.** **Phosph.**

M. AC.—*Ars.* **Bry.** *Lyc.* **M. ac.**

NATR.—**Calc.** **Caust.** *Graph.* **Kali.** **Lyc.** *N. mur.* **Puls.** *Sep.* **Sil.** *Spig.* Sulph.

N. MUR.—**Alum.** **Anac.** *Ars.* **Brom.** **Cann.** *C. veg.* *Chin.* *Creos.* *Kali.* *Natr.* **N. vom.** **Petr.** **Puls.** *Ruta.* **Spig.** **Vit.**

NITR.—**Calc.** *Ipec.*

N. AC.—**Agar.** *Asaf.* *Bell.* **Bov.** **Calc.** *Cann.* **C. veg.** *Con.* *Fluor.* **Graph.** **Hep.** **Kali.** **Lyc.** **Merc.** **Mezer.** **Petr.** *Puls.* *Rhus.* **Sep.** **Sulph.** *Thuj.*

N. MOSCH.—**Cocc.** **Ignat.** **N. vom.** **Sep.**

N. VOM.—*Acon.* **Agar.** *Ambr.* **A. mur.** **Ars.** **Asar.** **Aur.** **Bar.** **Bell.** **Calad.** **Calc.** **Caps.** **C. veg.** *Caust.* **Cham.** **Chin.** *Cocc.* *Coff.* *Colch.* **Con.** **Creos.** *Cupr.* *Dig.* **Dros.** **Dulc.** *Euphr.* *Graph.* **Guaj.** *Ignat.* **Ipec.** **Kali.** *Lach.* **Lyc.** **M. austr.** **Magn.** **Merc.** **Millef.** **Mosch.** **M. ac.** **N. mur.** **Op.** **Par.** **Petr.** **Phosph.** **Plumb.** *Puls.* *Rheum.* **Rhus.** *Selen.* **Sep.** **Sil.** *Stram.* *Sulph.* *Valer.*

OLEAND.—**Cocc.** *Vit.*

OP.—*Acon.* *A. tart.* **Bell.** **Brom.** **Camph.** **C. veg.** **Cic.** *Coff.* **Colch.** *Croc.* *Cupr.* *Dig.* **Hyosc.** *Ipec.* **Merc.** **Mosch.** *N. vom.* **Phosph.** **Ph. ac.** **Plumb.** **Stram.**

PAR.—*Jod.* **N. vom.** **Phosph.**

PETR.—**Agar.** *Ars.* *Calc.* **C. veg.** **Cham.** *Lyc.* **N. mur.** *N. ac.* **N. vom.** **Phosph.** **Puls.** *Sil.* **Sulph.** *Thuj.*

PHOSPH.—**Acon.** **Agar.** **Alum.** *Amm.* *Ars.* **Aur.** **Brom.** *Calc.* *Caust.* **Chin.** **Cina.** **Dig.** *Graph.* **Hell.** *Jod.* **Ipec.** *Kali.* **Lyc.** **Mosch.** **N. vom.** **Op.** **Par.** **Petr.** **Puls.** **S. corn.** *Sep.* **Sil.** **Stront.** **Veratr.** **Verb.**

PH. AC.—**Acon.** *Ars.* *Asaf.* *Bell.* *Calc.* *Chin.* **Cupr.** *Dig.* **Dulc.** *Hyosc.* **Ignat.** *Lach.* **Lyc.** **Merc.** **Op.** *Rheum.* **Rhus.** *Staph.* **Veratr.** *Zinc.*

4

PLAT.—**Asaf. Bell.** *Caust.* **Croc.** *Dig. Ignat.* **Lach. Men. Merc. Plumb. Puls. Sabad. Sabin. Stront. Vit.**

PLUMB.—*Alum. Ars. Bell.* **Chin.** *Hyosc.* **N. mur.** *N. vom.* **Op. Plat.** *Stram.* **Sulph.** *S. ac.*

PULS.—**Acon.** *Agar. Alum. Ambr.* **A. mur. A. crud.** *A. tart. Ap. Arn. Asaf. Aur.* **Bell. Bry.** *Calc.* **Cann. Canth. Caps. C. veg.** *Caust.* **Cham. Chel.** *Chin. Coff. Colch. Con.* **Cupr.** *Cycl. Dig.* **Dulc.** *Euph. Ferr.* **Graph. Ignat.** *Ipec.* **Kali. Lach. Led. Lyc. M. arct. Magn. Mang. Merc. Millef. Natr. N. mur. N. ac.** *N. vom.* **Petr.** *Phosph.* **Plat.** *R. bulb.* **Rheum.** *Rhus. Sabad.* **Sep.** *Sil.* **Spig. Stann.** *Sulph.* **S. ac. Valer. Verb. Vit.**

R. BULB.—*Bry. Puls.* **Staph. Sulph. Verb.**

R. SCEL.—**Ars. Puls. Veratr.**

RHEUM.—*Bell. Cham. Coloc.* **Magn.** *Merc.* **N. vom.** *Ph. ac. Puls.*

RHOD.—**Bry. Calc. C. an. C. veg.** *Caust.* **Clem. Merc. N. vom. Rhus. Sep.**

RHUS.—**Acon. A. mur.** *Ang.* **Arn. Ars.** *Bell.* **Bry.** *Calc. Caust.* **Cham. Cic.** *Clem. Coff.* **Dulc. Euph.** *Hep. Lyc.* **Merc.** *Mezer.* **N. ac. N. vom. Phosph. Ph. ac.** *Puls.* **Rhod. Samb. Sep. Sil.** *Sulph.* **Veratr.**

RUTA.—**Ignat.** *N. mur.*

SABAD.—**Plat.** *Puls.*

SABIN.—**Arn. Calc. Plat.**

SAMB.—**Arn.** *Ars.* **Chin. Rhus.**

SASSAP.—**Bell. Calc.** *Merc.* **Sulph.**

SCILL.—*Arn. Ars.* **Bry.** *Millef.*

S. CORN.—**Amm.** *Ars. Bell. Coloc.* **Phosph. Veratr.**

SELEN.—**Alum.** *Bry. Bov. Calc. Ignat.* **Merc.** *N. vom. Puls. Sep.* **Sulph. Thuj.**

SENEG.—*Arn. Bell. Bry.* **Stann.**

SEP.—**Acon. Agar. A. crud.** *A. tart.* **Ap.** *Ars.* **Asaf. Bar. Bell. Bry.** *Calc.* **C. veg. Caust. Chin. Clem.** *Creos.* **Cupr. Dros.** *Dulc.* **Euph.** *Graph. Hep. Lyc.* **M. mur. Men. Merc.** *Natr.* **N. ac. N. vom.** *Phosph.* **Puls. Rhod. Rhus. Selen. Sil. Sulph. Veratr. Vit.**

SIL.—*Agar.* **Ars. Bell.** *Bor.* **Calc.** *Caust.* **Cupr.** *Fluor.* **Graph. Hep. Jod. Kali. Lyc.** *Merc.* **Mezer. Natr. N. vom.** *Petr.* **Phosph.** *Puls.* **Rhus. Sep.** *Staph.* **Sulph.**

SPIG.—**Bism. Dig. Euph. Laur.** *Merc. Natr.* **N. mur. Puls. Veratr.**

SPONG.—*Brom. Dros.* **Hep. Jod.**

STANN.—**Ars. Chin.** *Lach.* **Puls. Seneg. Sulph. Valer.**

STAPH.—*Ars.* **Bism. Coloc.** *Merc. Ph. ac.* **R. bulb.** *Sil.* **Sulph. Thuj.**

STRAM.—*Bell.* **Cham. Cic. Hell., Hyosc. Ignat.** *N. vom.* **Op.** *Plumb.* **Veratr.**

STRONT.—**Phosph. Plat. Sulph.**

SULPH.—**Acon. Ambr. A. crud.** *Ap.* **Ars. Bell. Bor. Calc.** *C. veg.* **Caust.** *Cham.* **Chel.** *Chin.* **Coff.** *Creos.* **Dulc.** *Ferr.* **Graph. Hep. Jod. Merc. N. ac.** *N. vom.* **Petr. Puls. R. bulb. Rhus. Sassap. Selen. Sep. Sil. Stann. Staph. Stront.** *Thuj. Valer.* **Vit.**

S. AC.—**Ars. Chin. Dig. Ferr. Ipec.** *Plumb.* **Puls.**

TAR.—**Con. Kali. Puls. Valer.**

THUJ.—*Cann.* **C. an.** *Hep. Graph. Merc. N. ac. Petr.* **Puls. Selen. Staph.** *Sulph.*

VALER.—**Acon.** *Bell. Cham. Coff. Hyosc.* **Ignat. Merc.** *N. vom.* **Puls. Stann.** *Sulph.*

VERATR.—*Acon.* **Alum.** *Arn. Ars.* **Bry. Calc. Camph. C. veg. Chin. Cic. Cina.** *Coff.* **Cupr.** *Dros. Ferr. Hyosc. Ipec.* **Merc. Phosph. Ph. ac. S. corn. Sep. Spig. Stram.**

VERB.—**Ang. Mezer. Phosph. Puls. R. bulb.**

VIOL. OD.—**N. vom. Phosph.**

VIOL. TR.—**Bar. N. ac. Rhus.**

VIT.—**Calc. Con. Graph. Lyc. Merc. N. vom.** *Oleand.* **Puls. Rhod. Sep. Sulph.**

ZINC.—**Arn. Bar. C. veg.** *Euph.* **Hep. Ignat. Lach.** *Mgs. M. arct. M. austr.* **Merc.** *Ph. ac.*

www.ingramcontent.com/pod-product-compliance
Lightning Source LLC
La Vergne TN
LVHW021201120826
845150LV00011B/2338

* 9 7 8 1 4 1 8 1 9 4 6 5 9 *